GASTROPARESIS DIET COOKBOOK FOR BEGINNERS

A New solution pain,receive your fitness with this 365day nutritious recipes Plus 30day meal plan including appetizer and healthy recipe to stay safe today.

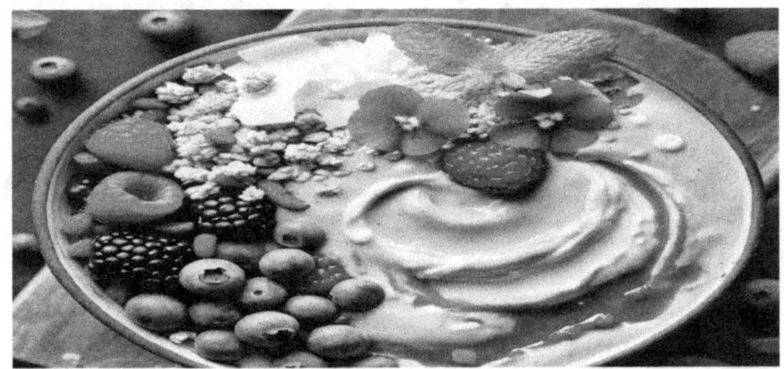

Dr. D. SAM

Copyright © 2024 Dr. D. SAM
Alright Reserved

Do not reproduce any of this book without
the permission of the copyright owner.

TABLE OF CONTENT

INTRODUCTION

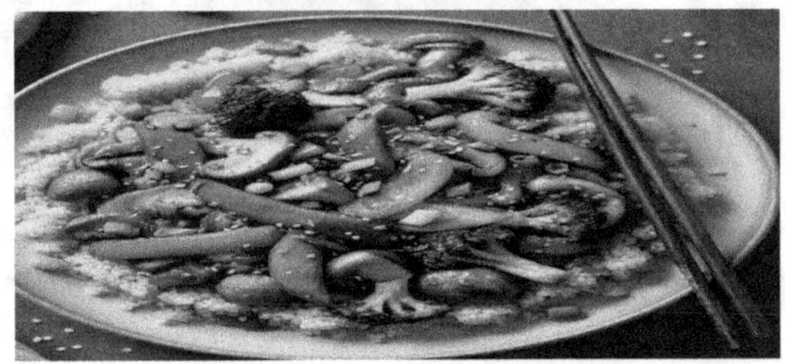

Welcome to the Gastroparesis Diet Cookbook for Beginners, your ultimate guide to managing gastroparesis with ease and confidence. Designed specifically for those new to the condition, this cookbook offers a curated collection of delicious and digestive-friendly recipes tailored to support your journey towards better health. With simple ingredients and easy-to-follow instructions, our cookbook empowers you to take control of your diet and discover a world of flavorful meals that nourish and satisfy. Say hello to a new chapter of wellness as you embark on this culinary adventure with us."

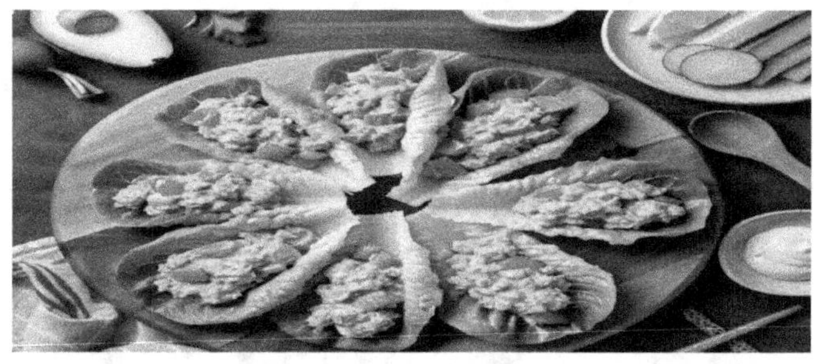

WHAT IS GASTROPARESIS?

Delayed stomach emptying is the hallmark of gastroparesis, a disorder that causes symptoms like bloating, nausea, vomiting, and a rapid feeling of fullness after eating. A dysfunction of the muscles or nerves that regulate the passage of food through the digestive tract is the cause of this delay in gastric emptying. Numerous things, such as diabetes, nerve injury, drugs, or surgery, can contribute to it. In order to reduce symptoms and enhance quality of life, managing gastroparesis usually entails dietary adjustments, drugs to aid in stomach emptying, and lifestyle changes.

FOODS TO EAT IN GASTROPARESIS

It's crucial to concentrate on foods that are simple to digest and unlikely to worsen symptoms if you have gastroparesis. The following foods are suggested:

Fruits with Low Fiber Content: Peaches, melons, and bananas.
Cooked Vegetables: Squash, potatoes, and carrots are examples of soft, cooked vegetables.
Lean Proteins: Fish, tofu, eggs, and skinless chicken are easier to digest.

Low-Fat Dairy: Opt for dairy products like cheese, yogurt, and milk that are low-fat or non-fat.

Grains: Refined grains, such as white pasta, bread, and rice, are preferable to whole grains.

Nut butter, avocado, and olive oil are examples of foods high in healthful fats that can be tolerated in moderation.

Clear soups and broths: These foods can supply nutrients without packing on the pounds.

Soft foods include things like oatmeal, mashed potatoes, and scrambled eggs that are simple to chew and swallow.

To assist with symptom management, don't forget to consume smaller, more often meals. Drinking liquids throughout the day is another vital way to stay hydrated. However, consuming a lot of liquids either before or right after a meal can make symptoms worse by adding to stomach emptying. For individualized nutritional guidance, speaking with a certified dietitian or other medical practitioner is also advised.

FOOD TO AVOID IN GASTROPARESIS

Certain foods should be avoided as they may aggravate symptoms of gastroparesis. The following foods should be avoided:

High-Fiber Foods: Berries, raw veggies, and whole grains can all be uncomfortable and difficult to digest.

High-Fat Foods: Rich sauces, fatty meat cuts, and oily or fried foods can all cause symptoms to intensify and prolong the emptying of the stomach.

Big Meals: Eating a lot of food can put a strain on the stomach and cause bloating, discomfort, and sensations of fullness.

Carbonated Drinks: Gas and stomach expansion brought on by carbonation might result in bloating and discomfort.

Alcohol: Consuming alcoholic beverages might worsen symptoms like nausea and vomiting and slow down digestion.

Foods that are spicy or highly seasoned: These foods might aggravate symptoms like nausea and heartburn by irritating the lining of the stomach.

Citrus Fruits: Because citrus fruits and juices, such oranges, grapefruits, and lemons, can be acidic, some people may have reflux or other discomfort.

Tough Meats: Meats with gristle and tough cuts of meat can be uncomfortable to chew and digest.

Sweets, desserts, and sugary drinks are examples of foods and beverages high in added sugar that can quickly alter blood sugar levels and exacerbate symptoms.

It's critical to pay attention to your body and stay away from foods that may aggravate or cause symptoms of gastroparesis. A customised nutrition plan that suits your individual requirements and tastes can be created by working with a healthcare expert or a qualified dietitian.

Banana Oatmeal

- Ingredients:
    1. 1/2 cup oats
    2. 1 cup water or low-fat milk
    3. 1 ripe banana, mashed
    4. Cinnamon (optional)
- Instructions:
    1. In a small saucepan, bring water or milk to a boil.
    2. Stir in oats and reduce heat to low. Cook for 5-7 minutes, stirring occasionally until oats are creamy.
    3. Mix in mashed banana and cook for an additional 1-2 minutes.
    4. Sprinkle with cinnamon if desired and serve warm.

Scrambled Eggs with Spinach

- Ingredients:
    1. 2 eggs
    2. 1/4 cup fresh spinach, chopped
    3. Salt and pepper to taste
    4. 1 tsp olive oil or cooking spray
- Instructions:
    1. In a bowl, beat eggs with salt and pepper.
    2. Heat olive oil or cooking spray in a non-stick skillet over medium heat.
    3. Add chopped spinach to the skillet and cook for 1-2 minutes until wilted.
    4. Pour beaten eggs into the skillet and cook, stirring gently, until eggs are set.
    5. Serve hot.

Yogurt Parfait

- Ingredients:
  1. 1/2 cup low-fat Greek yogurt
  2. 1/4 cup granola (choose a low-fiber option)
  3. 1/4 cup fresh berries (such as strawberries, blueberries, or raspberries)
  4. 1 tsp honey (optional)
- Instructions:
  1. In a glass or bowl, layer Greek yogurt, granola, and fresh berries.
  2. Drizzle with honey if desired.
  3. Repeat layers if desired.
  4. Serve immediately.

Smooth Peanut Butter Toast

- Ingredients:

1. 1 slice whole wheat bread (choose a low-fiber option)
2. 1 tbsp smooth peanut butter
3. 1/2 small banana, sliced
- Instructions:
1. Toast the slice of bread until golden brown.
2. Spread peanut butter evenly over the toast.
3. Top with sliced banana.
4. Enjoy as an open-faced sandwich.

Vanilla Chia Seed Pudding

- Ingredients:
1. 2 tbsp chia seeds
2. 1/2 cup low-fat milk or almond milk
3. 1/4 tsp vanilla extract
4. 1 tsp honey (optional)
- Instructions:

1. In a bowl or jar, mix chia
   seeds, milk, vanilla extract,
   and honey (if using).
2. Stir well to combine.
3. Cover and refrigerate for
   at least 2 hours or
   overnight, until the
   mixture thickens.
4. Serve chilled, optionally
   topped with fresh berries
   or sliced fruit.

Mashed Banana Pancakes

- Ingredients:
  1. 1 ripe banana, mashed
  2. 1 egg
  3. 1/4 tsp baking powder
  4. Cooking spray or oil for
     greasing
- Instructions:
  1. In a bowl, mix mashed
     banana, egg, and baking
     powder until well
     combined.

2. Heat a non-stick skillet or griddle over medium heat and lightly grease with cooking spray or oil.
3. Pour small portions of the batter onto the skillet to form pancakes.
4. Cook until bubbles form on the surface, then flip and cook until golden brown on both sides.
5. Serve warm with a drizzle of honey or maple syrup if desired.

Creamy Rice Pudding

- Ingredients:
    1. 1/2 cup cooked white rice
    2. 1/2 cup low-fat milk or almond milk
    3. 1/4 tsp vanilla extract
    4. 1 tsp honey (optional)
    5. Ground cinnamon for garnish

- ○ Instructions:
    1. In a small saucepan, combine cooked rice, milk, vanilla extract, and honey (if using).
    2. Cook over medium-low heat, stirring occasionally, until the mixture thickens to a pudding-like consistency.
    3. Remove from heat and let cool slightly.
    4. Serve warm or chilled, sprinkled with ground cinnamon.

Egg and Cheese Breakfast Muffins

- ○ Ingredients:
    1. 2 eggs
    2. 1/4 cup shredded low-fat cheese
    3. Salt and pepper to taste
    4. Cooking spray for greasing
- ○ Instructions:

1. Preheat the oven to 350°F (175°C) and grease a muffin tin with cooking spray.
2. In a bowl, whisk together eggs, shredded cheese, salt, and pepper.
3. Pour the egg mixture into the prepared muffin tin, filling each cup about halfway.
4. Bake for 15-20 minutes or until the muffins are set and lightly golden.
5. Allow to cool slightly before removing from the muffin tin. Serve warm.

Apple Cinnamon Rice Porridge

- Ingredients:
  1. 1/2 cup cooked white rice
  2. 1/2 cup unsweetened applesauce
  3. 1/4 tsp cinnamon

4. 1 tsp honey (optional)

- Instructions:
    1. In a small saucepan, combine cooked rice, applesauce, cinnamon, and honey (if using).
    2. Cook over low heat, stirring occasionally, until heated through.
    3. Serve warm, optionally topped with a sprinkle of additional cinnamon.

Yogurt and Berry Smoothie Bowl

- Ingredients:
    1. 1/2 cup low-fat Greek yogurt
    2. 1/4 cup fresh berries (such as strawberries, blueberries, or raspberries)
    3. 1 tbsp sliced almonds or chopped nuts
    4. 1 tsp honey (optional)

- ○ Instructions:
    1. In a bowl, spread Greek yogurt evenly.
    2. Top with fresh berries and sliced almonds or chopped nuts.
    3. Drizzle with honey if desired.
    4. Serve immediately and enjoy with a spoon.

LUNCH RECIPES

Chicken and Rice Soup

- ○ Ingredients:
    1. 1 boneless, skinless chicken breast
    2. 2 cups low-sodium chicken broth
    3. 1/4 cup cooked white rice
    4. 1 carrot, peeled and diced
    5. Salt and pepper to taste
- ○ Instructions:

1. In a pot, bring chicken broth to a boil.
2. Add chicken breast and diced carrot to the pot, reduce heat, and simmer until chicken is cooked through (about 15-20 minutes).
3. Remove chicken from the pot, shred it with a fork, and return it to the pot.
4. Add cooked rice to the pot and simmer for an additional 5 minutes.
5. Season with salt and pepper to taste before serving.

Turkey and Mashed Potato Bowl

- Ingredients:
  1. 1/2 cup cooked ground turkey
  2. 1/2 cup mashed potatoes

3. 1/4 cup steamed green beans
4. Gravy (optional)
- Instructions:
    1. Heat cooked ground turkey in a skillet until warmed through.
    2. Reheat mashed potatoes in the microwave or on the stovetop.
    3. Steam green beans until tender.
    4. Arrange the cooked turkey, mashed potatoes, and steamed green beans in a bowl.
    5. Serve with gravy on top if desired.

Tuna Salad Lettuce Wraps

- Ingredients:
    1. 1 can (5 oz) tuna, drained
    2. 1 tbsp mayonnaise
    3. 1/4 cup diced celery

4. Lettuce leaves for wrapping

- ○ Instructions:
    1. In a bowl, mix together drained tuna, mayonnaise, and diced celery.
    2. Spoon the tuna salad onto lettuce leaves.
    3. Wrap the lettuce around the tuna salad to form wraps.
    4. Serve immediately as a light and refreshing lunch option.

Egg Salad Sandwich

- ○ Ingredients:
    1. 2 hard-boiled eggs, chopped
    2. 1 tbsp mayonnaise
    3. 1 tsp mustard
    4. Salt and pepper to taste
    5. 1 slice whole wheat bread (choose a low-fiber option)

- ○ Instructions:
    1. In a bowl, combine chopped hard-boiled eggs, mayonnaise, mustard, salt, and pepper.
    2. Mix until well combined.
    3. Spread the egg salad onto the slice of bread to make a sandwich.
    4. Cut the sandwich in half or quarters for easier digestion.
    5. Serve with a side of cooked carrots or cucumber slices.

Vegetable Quinoa Bowl

- ○ Ingredients:
    1. 1/2 cup cooked quinoa
    2. 1/4 cup cooked diced chicken or tofu (optional)
    3. 1/4 cup steamed carrots
    4. 1/4 cup steamed zucchini
    5. 1 tbsp olive oil
    6. Salt and pepper to taste

- Instructions:
    1. In a bowl, combine cooked quinoa, diced chicken or tofu (if using), steamed carrots, and steamed zucchini.
    2. Drizzle olive oil over the quinoa bowl and season with salt and pepper to taste.
    3. Toss until everything is evenly coated.
    4. Serve warm as a nutritious and satisfying lunch option.

Salmon and Potato Hash

- Ingredients:
    1. 1 small salmon fillet, cooked and flaked
    2. 1 small potato, diced and boiled until tender
    3. 1/4 cup diced bell pepper
    4. 1/4 cup diced onion

5. 1 tsp olive oil
6. Salt and pepper to taste
- Instructions:
    1. Heat olive oil in a skillet over medium heat.
    2. Add diced bell pepper and onion to the skillet and cook until softened.
    3. Add cooked and diced potato to the skillet and cook until lightly browned.
    4. Stir in flaked salmon and cook until heated through.
    5. Season with salt and pepper to taste and serve warm.

Quinoa and Vegetable Stir-Fry

- Ingredients:
    1. 1/2 cup cooked quinoa
    2. 1/4 cup diced tofu or chicken (optional)
    3. 1/4 cup sliced mushrooms
    4. 1/4 cup diced bell pepper

5. 1/4 cup sliced zucchini
6. 1 tbsp low-sodium soy sauce
7. 1 tsp sesame oil

- Instructions:
    1. In a skillet or wok, heat sesame oil over medium-high heat.
    2. Add diced tofu or chicken (if using) and cook until lightly browned.
    3. Add sliced mushrooms, diced bell pepper, and sliced zucchini to the skillet and stir-fry until vegetables are tender.
    4. Stir in cooked quinoa and soy sauce, and cook until heated through.
    5. Serve hot as a flavorful and nutritious stir-fry option.

Turkey and Vegetable Soup

- Ingredients:

1. 1/2 cup cooked ground turkey
2. 2 cups low-sodium chicken broth
3. 1/4 cup diced carrots
4. 1/4 cup diced celery
5. 1/4 cup diced onion
6. Salt and pepper to taste

- Instructions:

1. In a pot, bring chicken broth to a boil.
2. Add diced carrots, celery, and onion to the pot and simmer until vegetables are tender.
3. Stir in cooked ground turkey and cook until heated through.
4. Season with salt and pepper to taste before serving.

Caprese Salad

- Ingredients:

1. 1 medium tomato, sliced
2. 1/4 cup fresh mozzarella cheese, sliced
3. 2-3 fresh basil leaves
4. 1 tsp olive oil
5. Balsamic glaze for drizzling (optional)

- Instructions:
   1. Arrange tomato slices and mozzarella cheese slices on a plate.
   2. Tuck fresh basil leaves between the tomato and cheese slices.
   3. Drizzle olive oil over the salad and balsamic glaze if desired.
   4. Serve as a light and refreshing salad option.

Greek Yogurt Chicken Salad

- Ingredients:
   1. 1/2 cup cooked chicken breast, diced

2. 1/4 cup diced cucumber
3. 1/4 cup halved cherry tomatoes
4. 2 tbsp plain Greek yogurt
5. 1 tsp lemon juice
6. Salt and pepper to taste

- Instructions:
    1. In a bowl, combine diced chicken breast, diced cucumber, and halved cherry tomatoes.
    2. In a separate bowl, mix together Greek yogurt and lemon juice.
    3. Pour the yogurt dressing over the chicken and vegetable mixture and toss until evenly coated.
    4. Season with salt and pepper to taste and serve chilled.

Baked Chicken and Mashed Sweet Potatoes

- o Ingredients:
    1. 1 boneless, skinless chicken breast
    2. 1 small sweet potato, peeled and diced
    3. 1 tsp olive oil
    4. Salt and pepper to taste
- o Instructions:
    1. Preheat the oven to 375°F (190°C).
    2. Place the chicken breast on a baking sheet lined with parchment paper.
    3. Drizzle olive oil over the chicken breast and season with salt and pepper.
    4. Bake in the preheated oven for 20-25 minutes or until cooked through.

5. Meanwhile, boil the diced sweet potato until tender, then mash until smooth.
6. Serve the baked chicken with mashed sweet potatoes on the side.

Salmon and Quinoa Salad

- Ingredients:
  1. 1 salmon fillet
  2. 1/2 cup cooked quinoa
  3. 1 cup mixed salad greens
  4. 1/4 cup cherry tomatoes, halved
  5. 1/4 cup cucumber, sliced
  6. 1 tbsp olive oil
  7. 1 tbsp lemon juice
  8. Salt and pepper to taste
- Instructions:
  1. Season the salmon fillet with salt and pepper and bake in a preheated oven at 375°F (190°C) for 15-20

minutes or until cooked through.
2. In a bowl, mix cooked quinoa, mixed salad greens, cherry tomatoes, and cucumber.
3. Drizzle olive oil and lemon juice over the salad and toss to combine.
4. Serve the baked salmon on top of the quinoa salad.

Turkey Meatballs with Tomato Sauce

- Ingredients:
    1. 1/2 lb ground turkey
    2. 1/4 cup breadcrumbs
    3. 1 egg
    4. 1/4 cup grated Parmesan cheese
    5. 1 cup tomato sauce
    6. 1/2 tsp Italian seasoning
    7. Salt and pepper to taste
- Instructions:

1. Preheat the oven to 375°F (190°C) and line a baking sheet with parchment paper.
2. In a bowl, mix together ground turkey, breadcrumbs, egg, Parmesan cheese, Italian seasoning, salt, and pepper until well combined.
3. Roll the mixture into meatballs and place them on the prepared baking sheet.
4. Bake in the preheated oven for 15-20 minutes or until cooked through.
5. Heat tomato sauce in a saucepan and serve the turkey meatballs with the sauce.

Vegetable Stir-Fry with Tofu

- Ingredients:

1. 1/2 block tofu, pressed and cubed
2. 1 cup mixed vegetables (such as bell peppers, broccoli, and carrots), sliced
3. 1 tbsp olive oil
4. 2 tbsp low-sodium soy sauce
5. 1/2 tsp ginger, minced
6. Cooked white rice for serving

- Instructions:
    1. Heat olive oil in a skillet over medium heat.
    2. Add cubed tofu to the skillet and cook until golden brown on all sides.
    3. Add sliced vegetables and minced ginger to the skillet and stir-fry until vegetables are tender-crisp.

4. Pour soy sauce over the tofu and vegetables and toss to coat.
5. Serve the vegetable stir-fry with cooked white rice.

Mashed Cauliflower with Grilled Chicken

- Ingredients:
    1. 1 boneless, skinless chicken breast
    2. 1/2 head cauliflower, chopped into florets
    3. 1 tbsp butter or olive oil
    4. Salt and pepper to taste
- Instructions:
    1. Season the chicken breast with salt and pepper and grill until cooked through.
    2. Meanwhile, steam or boil the cauliflower florets until tender.
    3. Drain the cauliflower and transfer it to a food processor.

4. Add butter or olive oil to the cauliflower and process until smooth.
5. Serve the mashed cauliflower with grilled chicken on top.

Tilapia with Steamed Vegetables

- Ingredients:
  1. 1 tilapia fillet
  2. 1/2 cup mixed steamed vegetables (such as carrots, zucchini, and green beans)
  3. 1 tsp olive oil
  4. Lemon wedges for serving
  5. Salt and pepper to taste
- Instructions:
  1. Preheat the oven to 375°F (190°C).
  2. Place the tilapia fillet on a baking sheet lined with parchment paper.

3. Drizzle olive oil over the tilapia and season with salt and pepper.
4. Bake in the preheated oven for 15-20 minutes or until the fish flakes easily with a fork.
5. Serve the tilapia with steamed vegetables on the side and lemon wedges for squeezing.

Turkey and Rice Soup

- Ingredients:
    1. 1/2 cup cooked ground turkey
    2. 2 cups low-sodium chicken broth
    3. 1/4 cup cooked white rice
    4. 1 carrot, peeled and diced
    5. 1 celery stalk, diced
    6. Salt and pepper to taste
- Instructions:

1. In a pot, bring chicken broth to a boil.
2. Add diced carrot and celery to the pot and simmer until vegetables are tender.
3. Stir in cooked ground turkey and cooked white rice, and cook until heated through.
4. Season with salt and pepper to taste before serving.

Eggplant and Tomato Bake

- Ingredients:
  1. 1 small eggplant, sliced into rounds
  2. 1 tomato, sliced
  3. 1/4 cup shredded mozzarella cheese
  4. 1 tbsp olive oil
  5. Italian seasoning for garnish

6. Salt and pepper to taste

- ○ Instructions:
    1. Preheat the oven to 375°F (190°C).
    2. Arrange eggplant slices on a baking sheet lined with parchment paper.
    3. Drizzle olive oil over the eggplant slices and season with salt and pepper.
    4. Top each eggplant slice with a slice of tomato and sprinkle with shredded mozzarella cheese.
    5. Bake in the preheated oven for 20-25 minutes or until the cheese is melted and bubbly.
    6. Sprinkle with Italian seasoning before serving.

Spinach and Feta Stuffed Chicken Breast

- ○ Ingredients:

1. 1 boneless, skinless chicken breast
2. 1/4 cup cooked spinach, squeezed dry
3. 2 tbsp crumbled feta cheese
4. Salt and pepper to taste
- Instructions:
    1. Preheat the oven to 375°F (190°C).
    2. Make a pocket in the chicken breast by slicing horizontally.
    3. Stuff the chicken breast with cooked spinach and crumbled feta cheese.
    4. Season the outside of the chicken breast with salt and pepper.
    5. Bake in the preheated oven for 25-30 minutes or until the chicken is cooked through.
    6. Slice and serve hot.

Shrimp Stir-Fry with Brown Rice

- Ingredients:
  1. 1/2 lb shrimp, peeled and deveined
  2. 1 cup mixed vegetables (such as bell peppers, snap peas, and carrots), sliced
  3. 1 cup cooked brown rice
  4. 1 tbsp low-sodium soy sauce
  5. 1 tsp sesame oil
  6. 1/2 tsp ginger, minced
- Instructions:
  1. Heat sesame oil in a skillet or wok over medium-high heat.
  2. Add shrimp to the skillet and cook until pink and opaque.
  3. Add mixed vegetables and minced ginger to the skillet and stir-fry until vegetables are tender-crisp.

4. Stir in cooked brown rice and soy sauce, and cook until heated through.

5. Serve hot as a flavorful and nutritious stir-fry option.

DESSERT RECIPES

Banana and Peanut Butter Smoothie

- o Ingredients:
    1. 1 ripe banana, peeled and sliced
    2. 1 tbsp smooth peanut butter
    3. 1/2 cup low-fat Greek yogurt
    4. 1/2 cup unsweetened almond milk
    5. Ice cubes (optional)
- o Instructions:
    1. In a blender, combine sliced banana, peanut butter, Greek yogurt,

almond milk, and ice cubes if using.

2. Blend until smooth and creamy.

3. Pour into a glass and serve immediately as a delicious and satisfying dessert option.

Baked Apples with Cinnamon

- Ingredients:
    1. 1 apple, cored and sliced
    2. 1/2 tsp cinnamon
    3. 1 tsp honey (optional)
- Instructions:
    1. Preheat the oven to 375°F (190°C).
    2. Place apple slices in a baking dish and sprinkle with cinnamon.
    3. Drizzle with honey if desired.

4. Bake in the preheated oven for 15-20 minutes or until apples are tender.
5. Serve warm as a comforting and naturally sweet dessert.

Chia Seed Pudding with Berries

- Ingredients:
  1. 2 tbsp chia seeds
  2. 1/2 cup unsweetened almond milk
  3. 1/4 tsp vanilla extract
  4. 1 tsp honey or maple syrup (optional)
  5. Fresh berries for topping
- Instructions:
  1. In a bowl or jar, mix chia seeds, almond milk, vanilla extract, and honey or maple syrup if using.
  2. Stir well to combine.
  3. Cover and refrigerate for at least 2 hours or

overnight, until the mixture thickens.

4. Serve chilled, topped with fresh berries.

Frozen Yogurt Bark

- o Ingredients:
    1. 1 cup low-fat Greek yogurt
    2. 1 tbsp honey or maple syrup
    3. 1/4 cup mixed berries, chopped
    4. 1 tbsp unsweetened shredded coconut (optional)
- o Instructions:
    1. Line a baking sheet with parchment paper.
    2. In a bowl, mix Greek yogurt and honey or maple syrup until well combined.
    3. Spread the yogurt mixture evenly onto the parchment paper.

4. Sprinkle chopped berries and shredded coconut evenly over the yogurt.

5. Place the baking sheet in the freezer for at least 2 hours or until the yogurt is frozen.

6. Once frozen, break the yogurt bark into pieces and serve cold.

Ginger Poached Pears

- Ingredients:
    1. 2 ripe pears, peeled and halved
    2. 2 cups water
    3. 1/4 cup honey
    4. 1-inch piece of fresh ginger, sliced
    5. 1 cinnamon stick
- Instructions:
    1. In a saucepan, combine water, honey, ginger slices, and cinnamon stick.

2. Bring the mixture to a boil, then reduce heat and simmer for 5 minutes.
3. Add pear halves to the saucepan and simmer for 10-15 minutes, or until pears are tender.
4. Remove pears from the poaching liquid and let cool slightly.
5. Serve warm or chilled, optionally drizzled with some of the poaching liquid.

Coconut Chia Pudding

- Ingredients:
  1. 2 tbsp chia seeds
  2. 1/2 cup coconut milk (unsweetened)
  3. 1/4 tsp vanilla extract
  4. 1 tsp honey or maple syrup (optional)

5. Unsweetened shredded coconut for garnish

  - Instructions:
    1. In a bowl or jar, mix chia seeds, coconut milk, vanilla extract, and honey or maple syrup if using.
    2. Stir well to combine.
    3. Cover and refrigerate for at least 2 hours or overnight, until the mixture thickens.
    4. Serve chilled, topped with unsweetened shredded coconut for garnish.

Baked Peach Slices

  - Ingredients:
    1. 1 ripe peach, sliced
    2. 1 tsp honey (optional)
    3. 1/4 tsp cinnamon
  - Instructions:
    1. Preheat the oven to 375°F (190°C).

2. Place peach slices in a baking dish and drizzle with honey if desired.
3. Sprinkle cinnamon over the peach slices.
4. Bake in the preheated oven for 15-20 minutes or until peaches are tender.
5. Serve warm as a simple and naturally sweet dessert.

Peanut Butter Banana Bites

- Ingredients:
    1. 1 banana, peeled and sliced into rounds
    2. 2 tbsp smooth peanut butter
    3. Unsweetened shredded coconut or chopped nuts for garnish (optional)
- Instructions:

1. Spread peanut butter onto one side of each banana round.
2. Optionally, sprinkle unsweetened shredded coconut or chopped nuts over the peanut butter.
3. Place another banana round on top to create a sandwich.
4. Repeat with remaining banana slices.
5. Serve immediately as a satisfying and protein-rich dessert.

Vanilla Yogurt with Berry Compote

- Ingredients:
    1. 1/2 cup low-fat vanilla yogurt
    2. 1/4 cup mixed berries (such as strawberries, blueberries, and raspberries)

3. 1 tsp honey or maple syrup (optional)

- Instructions:
    1. In a small saucepan, combine mixed berries and honey or maple syrup if using.
    2. Cook over low heat, stirring occasionally, until the berries break down and form a compote-like consistency.
    3. Let the berry compote cool slightly.
    4. In a serving bowl, layer vanilla yogurt and berry compote.
    5. Serve chilled as a refreshing and naturally sweet dessert option.

Frozen Banana Bites

- Ingredients:

1. 1 ripe banana, peeled and sliced into rounds
2. 2 tbsp smooth peanut butter or almond butter
3. Unsweetened shredded coconut or chopped nuts for garnish (optional)

- Instructions:
  1. Spread peanut butter onto one side of each banana round.
  2. Optionally, sprinkle unsweetened shredded coconut or chopped nuts over the peanut butter.
  3. Place another banana round on top to create a sandwich.
  4. Repeat with remaining banana slices.
  5. Transfer banana bites to a parchment-lined baking sheet and freeze until firm.

6. Serve frozen as a delicious and satisfying dessert.

SNACKS RECIPES

Apple and Almond Butter

- o Ingredients:
    1. 1 apple, sliced
    2. 2 tbsp almond butter (smooth or crunchy)
- o Instructions:
    1. Spread almond butter onto apple slices.
    2. Serve immediately as a satisfying and nutritious snack.

Yogurt Parfait

- o Ingredients:
    1. 1/2 cup low-fat Greek yogurt
    2. 1/4 cup granola (choose a low-fiber option)

3. 1/4 cup fresh berries (such as strawberries or blueberries)

- o Instructions:
    1. In a glass or bowl, layer Greek yogurt, granola, and fresh berries.
    2. Repeat layers as desired.
    3. Serve immediately as a delicious and protein-rich snack.

Cottage Cheese and Pineapple

- o Ingredients:
    1. 1/2 cup low-fat cottage cheese
    2. 1/2 cup fresh pineapple chunks
- o Instructions:
    1. Combine cottage cheese and pineapple chunks in a bowl.

2. Serve immediately as a simple and refreshing snack option.

Rice Cake with Avocado

- Ingredients:
    1. 1 rice cake (choose a low-fiber option)
    2. 1/4 ripe avocado, sliced
    3. Salt and pepper to taste
- Instructions:
    1. Top rice cake with sliced avocado.
    2. Sprinkle with salt and pepper to taste.
    3. Serve immediately as a crunchy and creamy snack.

Hard-Boiled Egg

- Ingredients:
    1. 1 hard-boiled egg
- Instructions:
    1. Peel and slice the hard-boiled egg.

2. Serve immediately as a protein-rich and portable snack.

Smooth Peanut Butter Oat Bites

- Ingredients:
    1. 1/2 cup smooth peanut butter
    2. 1/4 cup honey or maple syrup
    3. 1 cup old-fashioned oats
    4. 1/4 cup unsweetened shredded coconut (optional)
- Instructions:
    1. In a bowl, mix together peanut butter, honey or maple syrup, oats, and shredded coconut (if using) until well combined.
    2. Roll the mixture into small balls using your hands.

3. Place the balls on a plate or baking sheet lined with parchment paper.
4. Refrigerate for 30 minutes to firm up.
5. Serve chilled as a satisfying and energy-boosting snack.

Carrot Sticks with Hummus

- Ingredients:
    1. 1 medium carrot, peeled and sliced into sticks
    2. 2 tbsp hummus
- Instructions:
    1. Serve carrot sticks with hummus for dipping.
    2. Enjoy as a crunchy and nutritious snack option.

Cucumber and Cream Cheese Roll-Ups

- Ingredients:
    1. 1 small cucumber, peeled

2. 2 tbsp cream cheese (choose a low-fat option if desired)
3. Fresh dill or chives for garnish (optional)
- o Instructions:
  1. Using a vegetable peeler, slice the cucumber lengthwise into thin strips.
  2. Spread cream cheese onto each cucumber strip.
  3. Roll up the cucumber strips and secure with toothpicks if necessary.
  4. Garnish with fresh dill or chives if desired.
  5. Serve immediately as a refreshing and low-calorie snack.

Banana Slices with Sunflower Seed Butter

- o Ingredients:
  1. 1 banana, sliced

2. 2 tbsp sunflower seed butter

- ○ Instructions:
    1. Spread sunflower seed butter onto banana slices.
    2. Enjoy as a creamy and satisfying snack.

Rice Cake with Cottage Cheese and Berries

- ○ Ingredients:
    1. 1 rice cake (choose a low-fiber option)
    2. 2 tbsp low-fat cottage cheese
    3. 1/4 cup fresh berries (such as raspberries or blackberries)
- ○ Instructions:
    1. Spread cottage cheese onto the rice cake.
    2. Top with fresh berries.

3. Serve immediately as a light and protein-rich snack.

Ginger Lemon Tea

- Ingredients:
    1. 1-inch piece of fresh ginger, sliced
    2. 1 cup water
    3. 1/2 lemon, juiced
    4. Honey or maple syrup to taste (optional)
- Instructions:
    1. In a small saucepan, bring water and sliced ginger to a boil.
    2. Reduce heat and simmer for 5-10 minutes.
    3. Remove from heat and strain out the ginger slices.
    4. Stir in freshly squeezed lemon juice and sweeten

with honey or maple syrup if desired.

5. Serve warm as a soothing and digestive-friendly beverage.

Berry Smoothie

- Ingredients:
    1. 1/2 cup mixed berries (such as strawberries, blueberries, and raspberries)
    2. 1/2 banana, sliced
    3. 1/2 cup low-fat Greek yogurt
    4. 1/2 cup unsweetened almond milk
    5. Ice cubes (optional)
- Instructions:
    1. In a blender, combine mixed berries, banana slices, Greek yogurt, almond milk, and ice cubes if using.

2. Blend until smooth and creamy.
3. Pour into a glass and serve immediately as a refreshing and nutrient-rich beverage.

Coconut Water with Lime

- Ingredients:
    1. 1 cup coconut water
    2. 1/2 lime, juiced
    3. Mint leaves for garnish (optional)
- Instructions:
    1. In a glass, combine coconut water and freshly squeezed lime juice.
    2. Stir well to combine.
    3. Garnish with mint leaves if desired.
    4. Serve chilled as a hydrating and electrolyte-rich beverage.

Chamomile Tea with Honey

- Ingredients:
    1. 1 chamomile tea bag
    2. 1 cup hot water
    3. Honey to taste (optional)
- Instructions:
    1. Place the chamomile tea bag in a mug and pour hot water over it.
    2. Steep for 5-7 minutes.
    3. Remove the tea bag and sweeten with honey if desired.
    4. Stir well and serve warm as a calming and digestive-friendly beverage.

Pumpkin Spice Latte

- Ingredients:
    1. 1/2 cup unsweetened pumpkin puree

2. 1 cup unsweetened almond milk
3. 1/2 tsp pumpkin pie spice
4. 1/2 tsp vanilla extract
5. Stevia or sweetener of choice to taste (optional)

- Instructions:
    1. In a small saucepan, heat pumpkin puree, almond milk, pumpkin pie spice, and vanilla extract over medium heat.
    2. Stir until heated through and well combined.
    3. Sweeten with stevia or sweetener of choice if desired.
    4. Pour into a mug and serve warm as a comforting and seasonal beverage.

Cucumber Bites with Tuna Salad

- Ingredients:
    1. 1 cucumber, sliced into rounds
    2. 1 can (5 oz) tuna in water, drained
    3. 2 tbsp mayonnaise (choose a low-fat option if desired)
    4. 1 tbsp chopped celery
    5. Salt and pepper to taste
    6. Fresh dill or parsley for garnish (optional)
- Instructions:
    1. In a bowl, mix together drained tuna, mayonnaise, chopped celery, salt, and pepper until well combined.
    2. Place cucumber rounds on a serving platter.

3. Spoon a small amount of tuna salad onto each cucumber round.
4. Garnish with fresh dill or parsley if desired.
5. Serve immediately as a light and protein-rich appetizer.

Stuffed Cherry Tomatoes with Cottage Cheese

- Ingredients:
    1. 12 cherry tomatoes
    2. 1/2 cup low-fat cottage cheese
    3. 1 tbsp chopped chives or green onions
    4. Salt and pepper to taste
- Instructions:
    1. Slice the top off each cherry tomato and scoop out the seeds and pulp.
    2. In a bowl, mix together cottage cheese, chopped

chives or green onions, salt, and pepper until well combined.

3. Spoon a small amount of cottage cheese mixture into each hollowed-out cherry tomato.
4. Serve chilled as a refreshing and protein-packed appetizer.

Greek Yogurt Deviled Eggs

- Ingredients:
    1. 6 hard-boiled eggs
    2. 1/4 cup plain Greek yogurt
    3. 1 tsp Dijon mustard
    4. 1 tsp lemon juice
    5. Salt and pepper to taste
    6. Paprika for garnish (optional)
- Instructions:
    1. Peel and halve the hard-boiled eggs lengthwise.

2. Carefully remove the yolks and place them in a bowl.
3. Mash the egg yolks with a fork and mix in Greek yogurt, Dijon mustard, lemon juice, salt, and pepper until smooth.
4. Spoon the yolk mixture back into the egg white halves.
5. Garnish with a sprinkle of paprika if desired.
6. Serve chilled as a creamy and flavorful appetizer.

Caprese Skewers

- Ingredients:
  1. Cherry tomatoes
  2. Fresh mozzarella balls
  3. Fresh basil leaves
  4. Balsamic glaze for drizzling (optional)
  5. Toothpicks or skewers
- Instructions:

1. Thread one cherry tomato, one mozzarella ball, and one fresh basil leaf onto each toothpick or skewer.
2. Arrange the skewers on a serving platter.
3. Drizzle with balsamic glaze if desired.
4. Serve immediately as a colorful and delicious appetizer.

Vegetable Crudité with Hummus

- Ingredients:
    1. Assorted raw vegetables (such as carrots, celery, bell peppers, and cucumber), sliced
    2. Hummus for dipping
- Instructions:
    1. Arrange sliced raw vegetables on a platter.
    2. Place a bowl of hummus in the center of the platter.

3. Serve immediately as a crunchy and nutritious appetizer.

BONUS

Chicken and Rice Soup

- Ingredients:
    1. 1 boneless, skinless chicken breast
    2. 4 cups low-sodium chicken broth
    3. 1/2 cup cooked white rice
    4. 1 carrot, diced
    5. 1 celery stalk, diced
    6. Salt and pepper to taste
- Instructions:
    1. In a large pot, bring chicken broth to a boil.
    2. Add chicken breast, carrot, and celery to the pot.

3. Reduce heat and simmer for 20-25 minutes or until the chicken is cooked through.
4. Remove the chicken breast from the pot and shred it using two forks.
5. Return shredded chicken to the pot.
6. Stir in cooked white rice and season with salt and pepper to taste.
7. Simmer for an additional 5 minutes.
8. Serve hot as a comforting and nourishing soup.

Vegetable and Quinoa Soup

- Ingredients:
    1. 4 cups low-sodium vegetable broth
    2. 1/2 cup cooked quinoa
    3. 1 carrot, diced
    4. 1 celery stalk, diced

5. 1/2 cup frozen peas
6. 1/2 cup frozen corn kernels
7. Salt and pepper to taste

- Instructions:
    1. In a large pot, bring vegetable broth to a boil.
    2. Add diced carrot and celery to the pot and simmer for 10 minutes.
    3. Stir in cooked quinoa, frozen peas, and frozen corn kernels.
    4. Season with salt and pepper to taste.
    5. Simmer for an additional 5 minutes.
    6. Serve hot as a hearty and nutritious soup.

Tomato Basil Soup

- Ingredients:
    1. 4 cups low-sodium tomato soup

2. 1/4 cup chopped fresh basil
3. 1/4 cup heavy cream (optional)
4. Salt and pepper to taste
- Instructions:
  1. In a large pot, heat tomato soup over medium heat.
  2. Stir in chopped fresh basil.
  3. If using, add heavy cream to the soup and stir until combined.
  4. Season with salt and pepper to taste.
  5. Simmer for 5-10 minutes, stirring occasionally.
  6. Serve hot as a flavorful and creamy soup.

Butternut Squash Soup

- Ingredients:
  1. 4 cups low-sodium butternut squash soup
  2. 1/4 cup plain Greek yogurt

3. 1/4 tsp ground nutmeg

4. Salt and pepper to taste

- Instructions:

    1. In a large pot, heat butternut squash soup over medium heat.

    2. Stir in plain Greek yogurt and ground nutmeg until well combined.

    3. Season with salt and pepper to taste.

    4. Simmer for 5-10 minutes, stirring occasionally.

    5. Serve hot as a creamy and comforting soup.

Lentil Soup

- Ingredients:

    1. 4 cups low-sodium vegetable broth

    2. 1 cup dried lentils, rinsed and drained

    3. 1 carrot, diced

    4. 1 celery stalk, diced

5. 1/2 onion, diced
6. 2 cloves garlic, minced
7. 1 tsp ground cumin
8. 1/2 tsp paprika
9. Salt and pepper to taste
- Instructions:
  1. In a large pot, bring vegetable broth to a boil.
  2. Add dried lentils, diced carrot, diced celery, diced onion, minced garlic, ground cumin, and paprika to the pot.
  3. Reduce heat and simmer for 20-25 minutes or until lentils are tender.
  4. Season with salt and pepper to taste.
  5. Serve hot as a hearty and protein-rich soup.

<u>BONUS</u>

Steamed Carrots

- Ingredients:
    1. 2 large carrots, peeled and sliced
    2. Water for steaming
    3. Salt and pepper to taste
    4. Fresh parsley for garnish (optional)
- Instructions:
    1. Place carrot slices in a steamer basket set over a pot of boiling water.
    2. Cover and steam for 8-10 minutes or until carrots are tender.
    3. Remove from heat and season with salt and pepper to taste.
    4. Garnish with fresh parsley if desired.

5. Serve hot as a simple and nutritious side dish.

Roasted Sweet Potatoes

- Ingredients:
  1. 2 medium sweet potatoes, peeled and diced
  2. 1 tbsp olive oil
  3. 1/2 tsp garlic powder
  4. 1/2 tsp paprika
  5. Salt and pepper to taste
- Instructions:
  1. Preheat the oven to 400°F (200°C).
  2. In a bowl, toss diced sweet potatoes with olive oil, garlic powder, paprika, salt, and pepper until evenly coated.
  3. Spread sweet potatoes in a single layer on a baking sheet lined with parchment paper.

4. Roast in the preheated oven for 20-25 minutes or until sweet potatoes are tender and lightly browned.
5. Serve hot as a flavorful and satisfying side dish.

Sautéed Zucchini

- Ingredients:
    1. 2 medium zucchinis, sliced
    2. 1 tbsp olive oil
    3. 2 cloves garlic, minced
    4. Salt and pepper to taste
    5. Fresh basil leaves for garnish (optional)
- Instructions:
    1. Heat olive oil in a skillet over medium heat.
    2. Add minced garlic to the skillet and sauté for 1 minute until fragrant.
    3. Add sliced zucchini to the skillet and sauté for 5-7

minutes or until zucchini is tender.

4. Season with salt and pepper to taste.
5. Garnish with fresh basil leaves if desired.
6. Serve hot as a simple and delicious vegetable side dish.

Steamed Green Beans

- Ingredients:
    1. 2 cups green beans, trimmed
    2. Water for steaming
    3. Salt and pepper to taste
    4. Lemon wedges for serving (optional)
- Instructions:
    1. Place trimmed green beans in a steamer basket set over a pot of boiling water.

2. Cover and steam for 5-7 minutes or until green beans are crisp-tender.
3. Remove from heat and season with salt and pepper to taste.
4. Serve with lemon wedges for squeezing if desired.
5. Serve hot as a vibrant and nutritious side dish.

Mashed Butternut Squash

- o Ingredients:
    1. 1 medium butternut squash, peeled, seeded, and diced
    2. 1 tbsp butter or olive oil
    3. Salt and pepper to taste
    4. Fresh thyme leaves for garnish (optional)
- o Instructions:
    1. Place diced butternut squash in a pot and cover with water.

2. Bring to a boil and simmer for 15-20 minutes or until squash is tender.
3. Drain the cooked squash and transfer to a bowl.
4. Add butter or olive oil to the bowl and mash the squash until smooth.
5. Season with salt and pepper to taste.
6. Garnish with fresh thyme leaves if desired.
7. Serve hot as a creamy and comforting vegetable side dish.

30DAY MEAL PLAN

Day 1:

- **Breakfast:** Banana and Peanut Butter Smoothie
- **Lunch:** Greek Yogurt Chicken Salad (shredded chicken breast mixed with

Greek yogurt, diced cucumber, and cherry tomatoes)
- **Dinner:** Baked Salmon with Steamed Carrots
- **Snack:** Rice Cake with Almond Butter
- **Beverage:** Ginger Lemon Tea

Day 2:

- **Breakfast:** Chia Seed Pudding with Berries
- **Lunch:** Lentil Soup
- **Dinner:** Turkey and Vegetable Stir-Fry (ground turkey cooked with mixed vegetables)
- **Snack:** Greek Yogurt with Fresh Berries
- **Beverage:** Coconut Water with Lime

Day 3:

- **Breakfast:** Scrambled Eggs with Spinach and Tomatoes

- **Lunch:** Caprese Salad (sliced tomatoes, fresh mozzarella, and basil drizzled with balsamic glaze)
- **Dinner:** Quinoa Stuffed Bell Peppers
- **Snack:** Cucumber Slices with Hummus
- **Beverage:** Chamomile Tea with Honey

Day 4:

- **Breakfast:** Overnight Oats with Almond Milk and Sliced Banana
- **Lunch:** Turkey and Vegetable Soup
- **Dinner:** Baked Chicken Breast with Roasted Sweet Potatoes
- **Snack:** Cottage Cheese with Pineapple
- **Beverage:** Berry Smoothie

Day 5:

- **Breakfast:** Greek Yogurt Parfait with Granola and Berries

- **Lunch:** Chicken Caesar Salad (grilled chicken breast, romaine lettuce, cherry tomatoes, and Caesar dressing)
- **Dinner:** Vegetable and Quinoa Stir-Fry
- **Snack:** Rice Cake with Cottage Cheese and Berries
- **Beverage:** Pumpkin Spice Latte

Day 6:

- **Breakfast:** Banana Pancakes (made with mashed banana, eggs, and oats)
- **Lunch:** Tomato Basil Soup with Grilled Cheese Sandwich (using whole grain bread and low-fat cheese)
- **Dinner:** Baked Cod with Steamed Green Beans
- **Snack:** Apple Slices with Peanut Butter
- **Beverage:** Coconut Chia Pudding

Day 7:

- **Breakfast:** Spinach and Feta Omelette
- **Lunch:** Butternut Squash Soup with Whole Grain Crackers
- **Dinner:** Turkey Meatballs with Zucchini Noodles
- **Snack:** Carrot Sticks with Hummus
- **Beverage:** Green Tea with Lemon

Day 8:

- **Breakfast:** Greek Yogurt with Sliced Peaches
- **Lunch:** Quinoa Salad with Cucumber, Cherry Tomatoes, and Lemon Vinaigrette
- **Dinner:** Baked Chicken Thighs with Mashed Butternut Squash
- **Snack:** Rice Cake with Sunflower Seed Butter
- **Beverage:** Ginger Lemon Tea

Day 9:

- **Breakfast:** Smoothie Bowl with Mixed Berries, Greek Yogurt, and Granola
- **Lunch:** Lentil and Vegetable Soup
- **Dinner:** Grilled Salmon with Steamed Green Beans
- **Snack:** Apple Slices with Almond Butter
- **Beverage:** Coconut Water with Lime

Day 10:

- **Breakfast:** Oatmeal with Sliced Banana and Cinnamon
- **Lunch:** Spinach Salad with Grilled Chicken, Avocado, and Balsamic Vinaigrette
- **Dinner:** Turkey and Vegetable Stir-Fry with Brown Rice
- **Snack:** Cottage Cheese with Pineapple
- **Beverage:** Chamomile Tea with Honey

Day 11:

- **Breakfast:** Scrambled Eggs with Spinach and Feta Cheese
- **Lunch:** Greek Yogurt Chicken Salad (shredded chicken breast mixed with Greek yogurt, diced cucumber, and cherry tomatoes)
- **Dinner:** Baked Cod with Roasted Sweet Potatoes
- **Snack:** Carrot Sticks with Hummus
- **Beverage:** Berry Smoothie

Day 12:

- **Breakfast:** Chia Seed Pudding with Fresh Berries
- **Lunch:** Tomato Basil Soup with Whole Grain Crackers
- **Dinner:** Vegetable and Tofu Stir-Fry
- **Snack:** Rice Cake with Cottage Cheese and Berries
- **Beverage:** Pumpkin Spice Latte

Day 13:

- **Breakfast:** Greek Yogurt Parfait with Granola and Sliced Peaches
- **Lunch:** Turkey and Vegetable Soup
- **Dinner:** Baked Chicken Breast with Steamed Carrots
- **Snack:** Cucumber Slices with Hummus
- **Beverage:** Coconut Chia Pudding

Day 14:

- **Breakfast:** Banana Pancakes with Maple Syrup
- **Lunch:** Caprese Salad (sliced tomatoes, fresh mozzarella, and basil drizzled with balsamic glaze)
- **Dinner:** Turkey Meatballs with Zucchini Noodles
- **Snack:** Apple Slices with Peanut Butter
- **Beverage:** Green Tea with Lemon

Day 15:

- **Breakfast:** Greek Yogurt with Sliced Strawberries and Honey
- **Lunch:** Quinoa Salad with Cherry Tomatoes, Cucumber, and Lemon Vinaigrette
- **Dinner:** Baked Salmon with Steamed Asparagus
- **Snack:** Rice Cake with Almond Butter
- **Beverage:** Ginger Lemon Tea

Day 16:

- **Breakfast:** Smoothie Bowl with Mixed Berries, Greek Yogurt, and Granola
- **Lunch:** Lentil and Vegetable Soup
- **Dinner:** Grilled Chicken Breast with Mashed Butternut Squash
- **Snack:** Apple Slices with Almond Butter
- **Beverage:** Coconut Water with Lime

Day 17:

- **Breakfast:** Oatmeal with Sliced Banana and Cinnamon
- **Lunch:** Spinach Salad with Grilled Chicken, Avocado, and Balsamic Vinaigrette
- **Dinner:** Turkey and Vegetable Stir-Fry with Brown Rice
- **Snack:** Cottage Cheese with Pineapple
- **Beverage:** Chamomile Tea with Honey

Day 18:

- **Breakfast:** Scrambled Eggs with Spinach and Feta Cheese
- **Lunch:** Greek Yogurt Chicken Salad (shredded chicken breast mixed with Greek yogurt, diced cucumber, and cherry tomatoes)
- **Dinner:** Baked Cod with Roasted Sweet Potatoes
- **Snack:** Carrot Sticks with Hummus

- **Beverage:** Berry Smoothie

Day 19:

- **Breakfast:** Chia Seed Pudding with Fresh Berries
- **Lunch:** Tomato Basil Soup with Whole Grain Crackers
- **Dinner:** Vegetable and Tofu Stir-Fry
- **Snack:** Rice Cake with Cottage Cheese and Berries
- **Beverage:** Pumpkin Spice Latte

Day 20:

- **Breakfast:** Greek Yogurt Parfait with Granola and Sliced Peaches
- **Lunch:** Turkey and Vegetable Soup
- **Dinner:** Baked Chicken Breast with Steamed Carrots
- **Snack:** Cucumber Slices with Hummus
- **Beverage:** Coconut Chia Pudding

Day 21:

- **Breakfast:** Banana Pancakes with Maple Syrup
- **Lunch:** Caprese Salad (sliced tomatoes, fresh mozzarella, and basil drizzled with balsamic glaze)
- **Dinner:** Turkey Meatballs with Zucchini Noodles
- **Snack:** Apple Slices with Peanut Butter
- **Beverage:** Green Tea with Lemon

Day 22:

- **Breakfast:** Greek Yogurt with Sliced Strawberries and Honey
- **Lunch:** Quinoa Salad with Cherry Tomatoes, Cucumber, and Lemon Vinaigrette
- **Dinner:** Baked Salmon with Steamed Asparagus
- **Snack:** Rice Cake with Almond Butter
- **Beverage:** Ginger Lemon Tea

Day 23:

- **Breakfast:** Smoothie Bowl with Mixed Berries, Greek Yogurt, and Granola
- **Lunch:** Lentil and Vegetable Soup
- **Dinner:** Grilled Chicken Breast with Mashed Butternut Squash
- **Snack:** Apple Slices with Almond Butter
- **Beverage:** Coconut Water with Lime

Day 24:

- **Breakfast:** Oatmeal with Sliced Banana and Cinnamon
- **Lunch:** Spinach Salad with Grilled Chicken, Avocado, and Balsamic Vinaigrette
- **Dinner:** Turkey and Vegetable Stir-Fry with Brown Rice
- **Snack:** Cottage Cheese with Pineapple
- **Beverage:** Chamomile Tea with Honey

Day 25:

- **Breakfast:** Scrambled Eggs with Spinach and Feta Cheese
- **Lunch:** Greek Yogurt Chicken Salad (shredded chicken breast mixed with Greek yogurt, diced cucumber, and cherry tomatoes)
- **Dinner:** Baked Cod with Roasted Sweet Potatoes
- **Snack:** Carrot Sticks with Hummus
- **Beverage:** Berry Smoothie

Day 26:

- **Breakfast:** Chia Seed Pudding with Fresh Berries
- **Lunch:** Tomato Basil Soup with Whole Grain Crackers
- **Dinner:** Vegetable and Tofu Stir-Fry
- **Snack:** Rice Cake with Cottage Cheese and Berries
- **Beverage:** Pumpkin Spice Latte

Day 27:

- **Breakfast:** Greek Yogurt Parfait with Granola and Sliced Peaches
- **Lunch:** Turkey and Vegetable Soup
- **Dinner:** Baked Chicken Breast with Steamed Carrots
- **Snack:** Cucumber Slices with Hummus
- **Beverage:** Coconut Chia Pudding

Day 28:

- **Breakfast:** Banana Pancakes with Maple Syrup
- **Lunch:** Caprese Salad (sliced tomatoes, fresh mozzarella, and basil drizzled with balsamic glaze)
- **Dinner:** Turkey Meatballs with Zucchini Noodles
- **Snack:** Apple Slices with Peanut Butter
- **Beverage:** Green Tea with Lemon

Day 29:

- **Breakfast:** Greek Yogurt with Sliced Strawberries and Honey
- **Lunch:** Quinoa Salad with Cherry Tomatoes, Cucumber, and Lemon Vinaigrette
- **Dinner:** Baked Salmon with Steamed Asparagus
- **Snack:** Rice Cake with Almond Butter
- **Beverage:** Ginger Lemon Tea

Day 30:

- **Breakfast:** Smoothie Bowl with Mixed Berries, Greek Yogurt, and Granola
- **Lunch:** Lentil and Vegetable Soup
- **Dinner:** Grilled Chicken Breast with Mashed Butternut Squash
- **Snack:** Apple Slices with Almond Butter
- **Beverage:** Coconut Water with Lime

Discover the essential guide to managing gastroparesis with our comprehensive cookbook designed for beginners. Packed with easy-to-follow recipes and practical tips, our cookbook empowers individuals to navigate their gastroparesis journey with confidence. From nourishing soups to satisfying meals, our recipes are gentle on the stomach yet bursting with flavor. Say goodbye to uncertainty and hello to delicious, gastroparesis-friendly cooking. Take control of your health and embark on a journey towards wellness with our Gastroparesis Diet Cookbook for Beginners."

THE END

www.ingramcontent.com/pod-product-compliance
Lightning Source LLC
Chambersburg PA
CBHW050812250726
48653CB00006B/2184